Clinical Notes and the Patient Encounter

A Practical Guide for New Nurses on Thinking and Documenting Like a Healthcare Professional

Daniel Moir, BN

ISBN: 978-1-7642256-4-9

Dedication

This book is dedicated to my dear cousin Mattea Gill, whose enthusiasm for nursing inspired me to write it. If all new nurses are as curious and as eager to improve their practice as Mattea, the profession is in safe hands.

Clinical and Educational Disclaimer

This publication is intended as an educational resource only.

It does not replace local policies, organisational procedures, clinical guidelines, professional standards, legislative requirements, or independent clinical judgement.

Healthcare practices vary between jurisdictions and evolve over time. Readers must work within their scope of practice and comply with the policies and procedures applicable to their workplace, role, registration, and jurisdiction.

The examples contained in this book are provided to illustrate documentation principles and clinical reasoning. They are not intended to prescribe clinical procedures or override current workplace policy.

Clinical scenarios have been modified for educational purposes. Any resemblance to identifiable individuals is coincidental.

The author and publisher accept no responsibility for clinical decisions made solely on the basis of the information contained in this publication.

Contents

Introduction

During my nursing graduate year, like all new nurses, I often stayed back at the end of my shift to finish writing up my patient notes. I was slow. Painfully slow. Other, more experienced nurses would come past and kindly tell me to finish up and go home. I would usually reply that I was only slow because I was new, and that I would get faster soon.

And I did — but not in the way I first expected.

After my graduate year, I worked as a Community Nurse and later as a Clinical Nurse Educator (CNE). During my time as a CNE, I was asked to train six new nurses who had graduated from university and were beginning work in community nursing. Rather than focusing on clinical skills as individual care interventions, I found myself focusing on something broader — what I came to think of as the patient encounter.

The patient encounter encompasses everything that happens from the moment a patient and nurse begin a healthcare interaction, through to its completion — including how the encounter between them is documented afterwards.

For example, instead of simply teaching wound care, I would walk new nurses through the entire clinical care process: inviting the patient into the clinic, interacting with them, assessing the wound, performing the dressing, closing the encounter, and finally documenting what had occurred. The care and the notes were never separate things. They were part of the same process, regardless of the clinical setting.

On one occasion, a trainee nurse was typing up her notes while her computer screen was projected onto the wall so we could all see what she was writing. As she typed, she would record one part of the encounter, then jump back to add something she had just remembered, then move forward again, then backfill another detail. Notes that should have taken two to five minutes took closer to fifteen.

When she finished, the notes themselves were fine. They were accurate. Complete. But watching how she wrote them revealed something important.

First, she would not always have the luxury of fifteen minutes to write up the nursing notes for a single patient encounter. Fifteen minutes across four patients is an hour, and in any clinical setting, that delay quickly pushes everything way out.

Second — and more importantly — the way she wrote her notes reflected the way she had experienced the encounter itself. She moved from point to point because, in the moment, she had not been entirely sure how to approach the interaction or what her plan was. She had done the right things, but it was a little haphazard, without a clear internal roadmap.

I explained to her, and to the other nurses watching, that every patient encounter needs a plan — not a rigid script, but an understanding of how you are going to approach the patient interaction. I also explained that good nursing notes naturally reflect that process. When the encounter is clearer in your mind, the notes almost write themselves.

This book describes the process I used — consciously and unconsciously — in most patient encounters I had. It provides a simple roadmap for new nurses: how to enter an encounter, how to think during it, and how to document it clearly and efficiently afterwards.

Over time, I did become faster at writing my notes. But more importantly, I became more confident and more competent in my care. Do all nurses arrive at that space? I would say yes, but I often wish someone had taught me earlier about how to interact with a patient faster than experience eventually did. This book is my attempt to do that — to put into words what many nurses slowly develop over years of practice.

If this book helps you feel more confident in your patient encounters, clearer in your thinking, and more assured in your documentation, then it has done what it set out to do.

Policy First

My approach to the patient encounter developed over several years, shaped by experience, reflection, and the policies that governed my practice at the time I was working in community nursing and clinical nurse education. It evolved gradually, in response to real patients, real situations, and the realities of clinical care.

This book is not a textbook, and it does not replace local health policies, organisational procedures, professional standards, or scope-of-practice requirements. It is also not intended to prescribe a single "correct" way to practise nursing.

What this book offers is a structured way of thinking about the patient encounter and how that encounter can be documented clearly and safely. The examples and approaches described reflect how I learned to organise my thinking and my notes over time, within the frameworks and policies that applied to my own practice.

Healthcare settings differ. Policies change. What is appropriate in one organisation, jurisdiction, or clinical context may not be appropriate in another. If local policies, procedures, or clinical guidelines differ from anything described in this book, those policies and procedures must always take precedence.

This book should be read as a guide to thinking like a nurse, not a replacement for policy. It is intended to support nurses — particularly students and early-career practitioners — to approach patient encounters thoughtfully, to document their care clearly, and to practise safely within the systems in which they work.

Clinical judgement, scope of practice, and adherence to local policy remain the responsibility of the individual nurse.

Chapter 1: Before the Encounter

Very rarely Is a nurse required to provide care without first receiving some form of handover. At its core, handover exists to ensure continuity of nursing care. It is the mechanism by which responsibility for a patient is safely transferred from one nurse to another.

In an ideal world, every handover would be thorough, calm, and complete. In reality, handover can be chaotic. Patient load, time pressure, competing demands, and the need to complete routine nursing tasks - even fatigue - can all interfere with how information is recorded and shared. Over the course of my career, I have received handovers in many forms, from taped recordings to brief summaries, to detailed explanations outlining everything that occurred during the shift. Most were excellent and provided a clear clinical picture of the patient. Some, however, were not.

The poorest handover I have ever received happened in my first nursing year. It came from a paramedic who placed a patient in a room, handed me a manilla envelope as I entered the room, and hurried out the door. No explanation. No verbal summary. Just paperwork and a patient left in my care. I share this experience not to criticise, but to illustrate an important point: handover is not always reliable. When handover is incomplete or rushed, information can be lost. When information is lost, patient care can be compromised.

As a young nurse, I once received a handover in which I was told that a patient's blood pressure was low and needed to be increased if possible. No further information was provided. I knew that one simple way to support blood pressure was to encourage oral fluids, so throughout my shift I gave the patient regular glasses of water. I monitored his observations carefully, and by all measures, his blood pressure did improve.

However, towards the end of the shift I noticed that his legs and feet were swollen. When I gently pressed on the tissue, the indentations remained — a clear sign of pitted oedema. This swelling had not been present at the beginning of my shift. Concerned, I went back and reviewed the patient's notes more thoroughly. It was only then that I discovered the patient had known kidney impairment — information that had not been passed on at handover.

In trying to improve his blood pressure, I had given him more fluid than his kidneys were able to manage. I immediately reported this to the Nurse Unit Manager. A medical review was arranged, and the patient was prescribed Lasix. Although Lasix is often contraindicated in patients with impaired kidney function, in this case the patient's kidneys were still able to respond. He was transferred to the High Dependency Unit, and the outcome was ultimately positive.

Despite this, I felt awful. One of the core principles of nursing is to do no harm, and although my intentions were good, I had contributed to a clinical complication. That experience fundamentally changed my practice. From that day forward, I never relied solely on verbal handover again.

I made it a habit to read the patient's clinical notes — at minimum back to the most recent medical review — to get to know the patient more fully, familiarise myself with their nursing care plan, and look for any doctor's orders. I would then review the recent nursing notes to determine whether those orders had been completed. If they had not, implementing them became part of my care for that shift. If I was unable to do so, that information was clearly handed over to the next nurse.

Providing good nursing care involves far more than administering medications on time or ensuring patients have eaten and washed. An essential component of nursing care is understanding and carrying out medical orders. I once worked with a doctor who expressed frustration that a blood test he had ordered had still not been completed four days later. There was no clinical explanation documented — the order had simply not been followed. This delay compromised patient safety, as the results were needed to guide ongoing treatment.

Before entering a patient's room, it is important to take a few moments to understand who the patient is and what is happening with their care. This includes knowing their name, diagnosis, general clinical plan, and any information that may impact how you care for them during your shift. It would be impossible to provide a definitive list of everything that must be known, as what matters is often patient-specific. Experience teaches you what information is essential.

A useful guide is this: if a piece of information helps you care for a patient better, it will likely help another nurse do the same. As a student nurse, I once cared for a patient with advanced multiple sclerosis who became agitated during care. I discovered that gently rubbing her elbows helped calm her significantly. I made sure this information was handed over so that others could care for her more effectively.

Throughout a patient's healthcare journey, they will usually be cared for by many nurses across different shifts. While continuity is sometimes possible, changes in staffing due to illness, leave, or rostered days off mean that no nurse can assume they will care for the same patient from admission to discharge. This makes accurate handover and thorough preparation essential.

The key message of this chapter is simple: before you enter the room, take the time to understand as much about the patient's care as you reasonably can. Listen to handover, but do not rely on it alone. Read the patient's notes. Identify medical orders and ensure they are carried out. Any additional insights you gain should be documented and handed over so that care remains safe and consistent.

Documenting This

Although this was less common in community health settings, it can be useful to begin your shift documentation with a simple entry such as:

1415	Patient handed over.

This brief note establishes when responsibility for the patient's care was assumed. From that point until handover at the end of your shift, responsibility rests with you.

Once you have reviewed the available information and clarified the patient's plan of care, you are ready to meet the patient.

Please note that the times used in this and other examples in this book are for illustrative purposes only. I have recorded them in 24-hour time. Either 24-hour time or standard time is acceptable, but check your local health policies.

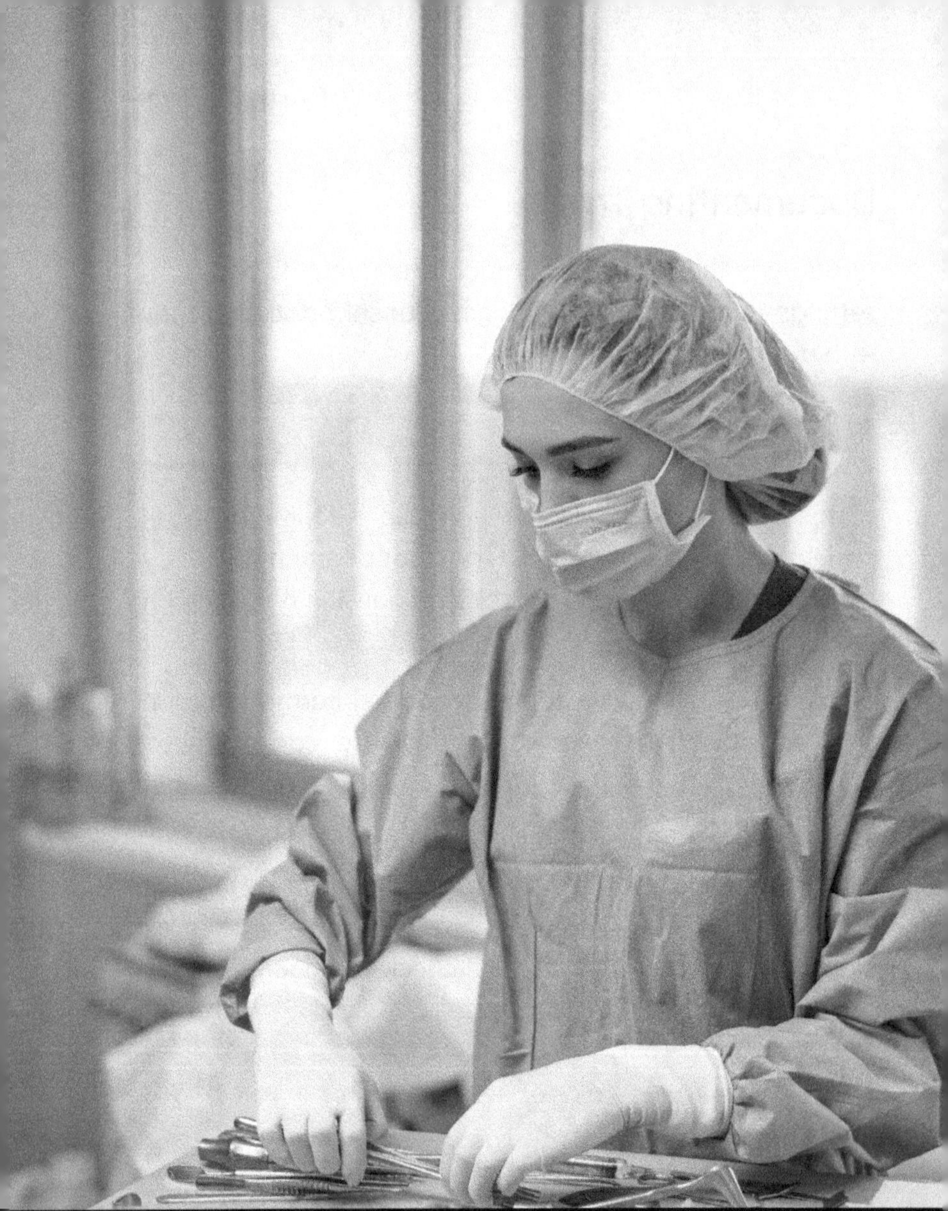

Practise safely and document what you do. Doing so helps protect your patients and your registration.

Chapter 2: The Patient Encounter

The Immediate Assessment

1006	Pt resting in bed. Alert and oriented. Normal breathing. No pain. Mood is good. Attending to ADLs.

The nursing encounter begins the moment the patient is committed into your care. That may occur at handover, during a home visit, or when a patient attends a clinic appointment. Regardless of the setting, the nurse's first priority is always the same: a rapid nursing assessment of the patient.

At the very beginning of any encounter, you are instinctively assessing for a medical emergency — or the potential for one. This happens quickly and often without conscious effort, particularly as your experience grows.

My first sentence in the nursing notes records where and how I encountered the patient. If I found the patient on the ward, I might write "Pt resting in bed". If the patient attended a clinic appointment, I would write "Pt attended clinic". If I found the patient after a collapse, I would write "Pt lying on the floor".

This opening sentence sets the scene for everything that follows. It anchors the encounter in place and context.

The following discussion is included to illustrate the importance of recognising and responding to immediate clinical deterioration. Basic Life Support requirements may change over time and may differ between workplaces and jurisdictions. Always follow the BLS protocol mandated by your employer, local health service, and current training.

The Vital Bit!

Your highest priority and concern in nursing is whether a patient needs immediate medical attention. If you do find a patient lying on the floor, or unresponsive in ANY manner, the absolute FIRST thing to do is to FOLLOW THE BASIC LIFE SUPPORT (BLS) ALGORITHM:

D - Check for Danger to yourself or to the patient

R - Check the patient for a response

If there is no response,

SEND FOR HELP IMMEDIATELY

Sending for help usually means hitting the Emergency Call button on the wall in the patient's room. However, it can also mean yelling for help at the top of your lungs if the button isn't readily available.

Then apply PPE, note the time, and:

A - Check the patient's airway. If you can easily remove any obvious obstruction, do so.

B - Check if the patient is breathing

If the airway is blocked and/or breathing is absent, start:

C - Chest compressions with rescue breaths as per your local health service protocol

D - When help arrives, direct them to get the defibrillator. When they return, have them attach the defibrillation pads to the patient's chest as per the instructions. The person attaching the pads works around the nurse doing the compressions to place the pads. Do not stop the compressions! Turn the defibrillator on, then, follow its instructions.

Continue this cycle until more advanced care arrives.

Continuing with Care

If there is no immediate medical intervention needed, what follows next is an initial nursing assessment:

0742	Alert and oriented. Normal breathing. No pain. Mood is good. Attending to ADLs.

This format is deliberate. It broadly mirrors the information captured on a Standard Adult General Observation (SAGO) chart, which is used in many Australian healthcare services. While other jurisdictions may use different observation charts, the underlying principles are largely the same.

In Australia, observation charts are often colour-coded, with yellow and red zones indicating increasing clinical concern. This system is commonly referred to as "Between the Flags" — a reference to the yellow and red flags used by surf lifesavers on Australian beaches to mark the safest area for swimming. If a patient's observations fall between the flags, they are generally considered stable. Patient instability occurs when observations trend toward the yellow or red zones.

A SAGO chart begins with airway and breathing, including respiratory rate and oxygen saturation. It then moves to circulation, recording blood pressure and heart rate. Disability follows, providing a brief neurological assessment — whether the patient is alert and oriented to their surroundings. Temperature and pain assessment are recorded next.

By writing in my clinical notes:

0742	Alert and oriented. Normal breathing. No pain. Mood is good. Attending to ADLs.

I am covering these same domains empirically — through observation and interaction rather than clinical numbers alone.

If a patient is alert and oriented, in a good mood, and not experiencing pain, there is no immediate neurological or pain-related emergency. If they are breathing normally, airway and breathing are adequate. If they are attending to their activities of daily living, circulation must also be sufficient. If any of these elements are abnormal, that signals the need for more immediate investigation or intervention.

I recall an experience early in my graduate year when I entered a patient's room to check on her. She was breathing rapidly and leaning forward, using her arms to support herself. I quickly assessed her breathing. Her respiratory rate was 33 breaths per minute. A healthy adult at rest typically breathes around 16 times per minute. This patient was clearly in respiratory distress.

That situation needed to be addressed promptly, before it became a full medical emergency. She was administered Salbutamol via nebuliser and given high-flow oxygen. Her breathing soon returned to normal.

When I was studying nursing, one of my tutors — an American ex-Navy nurse — offered a simple but enduring rule of thumb in clinical assessment:

"If air is going in and out and blood is going 'round and 'round, it's not a medical emergency."

Conversely, it **is** a medical emergency if blood is not going "round and round" — or is going round and out! Blood loss, of course, depends on volume. A small cut is not an emergency. A severed artery is.

Similarly, if air is going in and out but breathing is too fast, too shallow, or laboured while at rest, this may indicate that air is not effectively going in and out. My approach to the initial assessment of any patient has been strongly shaped by this way of thinking. If air is going in and out and blood is going ‘round and ‘round, then we usually have time.

> As a nurse, I have had many opportunities to interview student nurses for graduate positions at a rural New South Wales hospital in Australia. Inevitably, they were all asked what they would do if they found an unresponsive patient. It surprised me how many student nurses, hopeful for a graduate position, answered that question by stating that they would do a “Primary Survey”. When that happened, I would thank them for their answer and ask if they could go through the steps for me. Many stumbled, not knowing what to do. They knew the buzzwords. What they didn’t understand is what to do for an unresponsive patient.
>
> Knowing this is important because not only will it inform your nursing care, it will also set you apart from those who profess to know what they are doing, but do not. When I started at a rural hospital in NSW, there were nine nursing students applying for seven graduate nurse positions, so the chances were that I was going to be accepted. Within four years, there were 55 hopeful nurse students applying for the same seven openings.

A primary survey is a tool to assess and manage a patient in an emergency situation. It follows the Basic Life Support algorithm outlined previously in this chapter. Always follow your local health policies and procedures.

One of the things practical experience teaches a nurse is that you don't often notice things when they happen normally — unless you are actively looking for them. On one occasion, I was attending a presentation with a group of people when I noticed that one of the presenters was breathing heavily at rest. I watched for any sign of improvement for a little while. When none came, I interrupted gently and said something along the lines of, "My nurse's sense is tingling — are you all right?"

Nothing dramatic happened, but something important was noticed.

Healthy people do not usually breathe heavily while sitting quietly. Nor do they generally have a vague "unwell" appearance without reason. If you notice something out of the ordinary, investigate it further. Follow your nurse's sense. It will not take long to develop, and it is a vital part of clinical judgement.

For example, my father was admitted to hospital for a hip replacement post fall. Although the surgery had gone as planned, after a few days his condition deteriorated. After repeated interventions failed to improve his condition, I advocated for him to be transferred from Orthopaedics to Intensive Care. He received more direct care and my sister-in-law, herself an extremely talented sonographer, stopped in to see him one morning, after his treatment. She sent us a picture of his observations monitor. I reported to my mother that Dad's observations were looking excellent and, excitedly, we quickly drove to the hospital to see him. We walked into his room, I took one look at him, turned to my mother and said, 'I am so sorry, mum, but that patient does not match those obs.' Within half an hour, he started to deteriorate again and died a few days later.

In returning to clinical examination, you may also notice that my initial assessment does not always explicitly include exposure or temperature. That does not mean these are ignored. If a patient looks unwell, a full set of observations should be taken. If a patient reports chills or appears febrile, their temperature should be checked for confirmation.

This initial assessment does not take long when there is no medical emergency, but it is foundational to the entire patient interaction. By documenting it, you demonstrate how you found the patient, that the patient was not in immediate danger, and what you observed about their general condition at that moment.

Once the initial assessment has been completed, and you are satisfied that no immediate medical intervention is required, it is time to move on to the reason for the patient encounter.

When I reach this point in the encounter, I document the reason for the visit. In an example used in this chapter, the patient is attending the community health clinic for wound care. This can be recorded very simply by writing:

> For wound care.

If the patient is resting in a ward bed and I was there to take their observations, I would write:

> For obs.

That brief statement marks an important transition. Up until this point, the focus has been on safety, orientation, and general patient assessment. By documenting the reason for the visit, you signal that the encounter has shifted from initial assessment to task-specific care.

Documenting This

At this stage of the encounter, documentation serves a specific purpose: to record **how the patient was first encountered**, what was observed about their **general condition**, and whether there was any **immediate clinical risk**.

Clear documentation here reassures anyone reading the notes that the patient was stable at the time of assessment and provides a solid foundation for the care that follows.

Example: routine community health clinic visit

0742	Pt attended clinic. Alert and oriented. Normal breathing. No pain. Mood is good. Attending to ADLs.

This entry records orientation, stability, and functional ability, demonstrating that there was no immediate medical emergency.

Example: patient on ward in bed

0815	Pt resting in bed. Alert and oriented. Normal breathing. No pain. Mood is good. Attending to ADLs within limits.

Here, the documentation establishes context and stability while appropriately qualifying functional status.

Example: patient appearing unwell

0930	Pt attended clinic. Alert + oriented. Normal breathing. No pain. Mood appropriate. Attending to ADLs. Pt looks unwell. Asked if pt was all right. Pt replied he was. Obs taken as charted. Within acceptable parameters.

This entry shows that a concern was identified, investigated, and documented factually — without assumption or diagnosis.

Example: patient found collapsed on the floor and unresponsive

1137	Pt found on floor. BLS protocol activated. No apparent danger to pt or staff. No pt response. Emergency button pushed. PPE applied and time noted. Pt airway patent. No breathing.
1137	Compressions started as per BLS protocol.
1138	RN Black arrived. Told to get defib. Compressions continued as per BLS protocol.
1139	RN Black returned with defib. Pads placed on pt and pt monitored. Shock delivered and compressions resumed.
1140	Met team arrived. Pt handed over.

When I was nursing, BLS was an accepted abbreviation for Basic Life Support.

Here, the nurse records that the patient was found on the floor and the BLS protocol was enacted. It records that the nurse checked for danger and a response from the patient. When none happened, the emergency call button was activated, PPE was donned and the time noted. The patient's airway was checked as was their breathing before compressions commenced. If the patient was breathing but unresponsive, then the correct procedure - at least when I was nursing - is to place the patient in the recovery position and monitor until help arrives.

Example: rewrite of the poor handover mentioned in the previous chapter

0230	Pt handed over by paramedic. Pt resting in Room 1 bed 2. Alert and oriented. Normal breathing. No pain. Mood is good. Attending to ADLs within the limit of the pt's condition.

Here, there is no mention of the poor handover. That is because it matters little how poor the handover was in terms of clinical review if there is a review for an adverse patient event. When you receive care - however you received the care - you are now the nurse responsible for that patient. If you feel that something needs to be said about the handover, you can speak to the nurse in charge or nurse unit manager later. For now, though, the handover quality is unimportant. In terms of review for an adverse outcome, the reviewers will be interested in who was the nurse responsible for the patient at the time the event occurred.

Notice also that the patient's current location is recorded. This is because in a busy hospital, patients can be moved around to other rooms or wards as needed. A record of where the patient is when they arrive on the ward is important. Any change to a patient's location, if they are transferred to another room, should also be documented. This can be as simple as:

> Pt T/F to room 4 bed 1 at 1215. Clerk request.

At the time I was nursing T/F was an accepted abbreviation for ‘transferred’.

This records not only the fact that the patient was moved but on whose direction. If the patient required any ongoing monitoring, oxygen or other such equipment as part of their care, you need to record that these were reconnected and functioning. More will be said about this in the chapter on Incidental Care Notes.

At this point, documentation remains brief and focused. Detailed examination findings and interventions belong to the next stage of the encounter, which is explored in the chapters that follow.

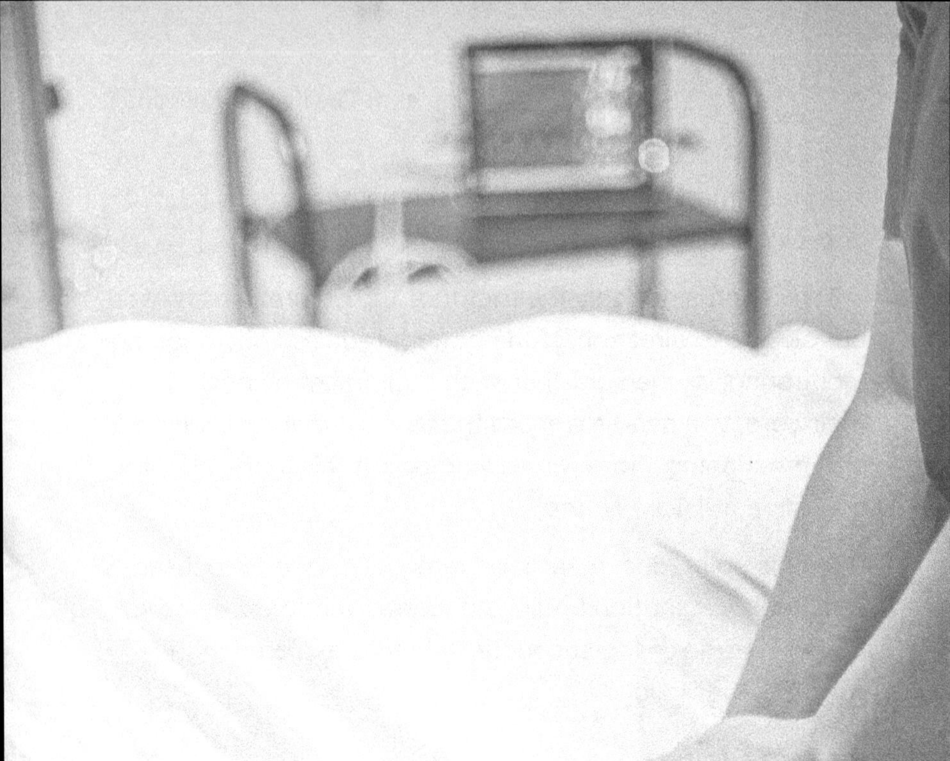

Always be kind to your patients. It makes a huge difference in care quality.

Remember: patient first, process second.

Chapter 3: On Examination

Once you have established that the patient is medically stable and you understand the reason for the encounter, you move into the next care phase — examination.

Most patient encounters involve a problem of some kind. To address that problem, you first need to understand what it is. That understanding does not come from assumptions or labels. It comes from looking carefully.

Looking Before Acting

Early in my community health practice, I was allocated a patient who was receiving wound care twice a week. When I arrived, I noticed that the limb with the wound was red and warm to the touch. Even with very little experience at that stage, something about it concerned me. My **nurse's sense** was activated.

At the same time, the patient herself was alert and oriented, breathing normally, in no pain, and attending to her activities of daily living. There was no immediate medical emergency. We had time.

I advised her that the limb looked red and swollen and recommended she see her GP. She did so, and later that week at my return visit, she told me she was diagnosed with cellulitis – a common complication in wound care – and had commenced antibiotics.

The important point here is not the diagnosis. It is that careful examination, paired with an awareness of the patient's overall stability, allowed the situation to be identified early and managed appropriately.

The Nurse's Sense

Throughout this chapter, you will see me refer to what I call my **nurse's sense**. As someone who enjoys science fiction and superheroes, I think of it as similar to Spider-Man's spider sense. His spider sense warns him when something isn't quite right.

Empirically, I define it as the sum of your nursing education and experience, subconsciously applied to assess a given healthcare situation. You may not always be able to articulate exactly why something feels "off" at first – but ignoring that feeling is rarely wise.

The good news is that your nurse's sense develops quickly. Every encounter you have sharpens it.

Seeing the Whole Patient

Observation is not confined to the specific reason for the visit. It must always include the patient as a whole.

I recall visiting a patient with a nursing student. The patient was resting in bed and receiving wound care. When I asked the student what she noticed, she initially said that the patient seemed to be resting comfortably. I asked her to look again — this time at his hands, and then at his feet.

His hands were pale white. His feet were deep purple.

Once she saw it, she immediately recognised that this was not normal. The patient was roused gently, spoke with us, and was alert and oriented, breathing normally, and in no pain — but the discrepancy in colour was an important finding that required further attention.

This kind of observation comes from slowing down just enough to really look.

Avoiding Tunnel Vision

Examination is not a rigid step that you complete once and move on from. It continues throughout the encounter.

As a Clinical Nurse Educator, I once supervised two new community nurses providing wound care to a patient with bilateral leg ulcers. Each nurse worked diligently on one leg, repositioning the patient as they focused on their individual tasks.

What they missed was the patient himself.

He was clearly uncomfortable, with his legs being manipulated in opposing directions. I asked the nurses to pause and reminded them that while technical care matters, they were caring for a person, not just wounds.

The patient was gracious about the situation, and the moment became a valuable learning experience.

Nursing care must never be so task-focused that you lose sight of the person in front of you.

Using All Your Senses

Observation is not limited to sight. Touch, hearing, and smell are all valuable tools in examination.

Touch, in particular, is often underused. With patient consent, it can provide vital information.

I once examined a patient following knee replacement surgery whose wound had dehisced. In the wound bed centre was a fibrous, purulent mass about the size of a large coin. The patient reported no pain. With consent and careful technique, I palpated the mass and realised it could be gently separated from the wound bed. I removed it without causing discomfort. There was no bleeding, and healing progressed rapidly afterwards.

In another instance, I was asked to assess a wound that appeared extensive. On examination, the problem turned out not to be an active wound at all, but a large accumulation of dry, dead skin. Once removed, only a small scab remained. There were no signs or symptoms of infection. The patient was admitted and discharged from care the same day.

Hearing can also be critical. During a student placement in Emergency, a patient arrived on an ambulance stretcher, sitting upright. He was breathing heavily. An experienced nurse quietly said to me, "Watch this patient. He's going to crash." Another experienced nurse also came up to me and said, "Watch this one."

They had noticed something I, and the other Emergency nurses attending to the patient hadn't — the absence of audible airflow. You would expect to hear the air rushing in and out from his exertion yet there was no sound at all. The patient was exhausted and struggling to breathe yet unable to draw air in effectively. Within minutes, he deteriorated and required urgent intervention.

Smell, too, can be diagnostic. On one occasion during a routine home visit, an elderly patient with an indwelling catheter had an overwhelming purulent odour in her room. On examination, her catheter bag contained white, foul-smelling discharge. Although she was initially stable, the findings warranted immediate escalation, and she was transferred to hospital. Interestingly, when the ambulance officers arrived, the one who entered the house first, before he even saw the patient, said: "This one is going to hospital." He could smell the purulent odour from the front door.

If something smells wrong, sounds wrong, or feels wrong — investigate it.

Gathering Evidence Before Acting

The purpose of assessment is to gather as much empirical information as possible. You are building a clinical picture based on what you can see, feel, hear, and smell — not what you assume.

This information:

- informs your clinical judgement
- guides your next steps
- supports safe decision-making

Equally important, it must be documented clearly and factually.

For now, the key point is this:

Assessment is about understanding what is happening — before deciding what to do.

Once you have assessed the patient, gathered your observations, and formed a clear picture of the situation, you are ready to move on to the next stage of care.

Documenting This

At this stage of the encounter, your documentation focuses on what you found on examination. The aim is to clearly and factually record your observations using neutral, descriptive language.

This is not the place for diagnosis or speculation. It is the place to document:

- what you saw
- what you felt
- what you heard

- what you smelt
- what the patient reported

When written well, these notes allow another clinician to clearly picture the patient and the health issue without having been present.

A General Principle

Begin by documenting how the area or issue was encountered, then move into a structured description. Avoid emotive or interpretive language. Let the observations speak for themselves.

Example: examination revealing no ongoing wound

> O/E:
> Skin to lower limb dry with extensive dead flaking skin. No open wound evident. Dead skin gently removed. Small scab present. No discharge. No odour. Surrounding skin intact No signs or symptoms of infection.

When I was nursing, O/E was an acceptable shorthand for 'On Examination'. This documentation shows that:

- the initial concern was explored
- examination altered the understanding of the problem
- unnecessary ongoing care was avoided

Example: wound examination (community setting)

> Dressings intact. Previous dressings removed. Some strikethrough noted. Surrounding skin healthy and intact.
>
> O/E:
>
> Wound located on left knee, post-surgical. Wound dehisced and measures approximately 5 cm in length and 3 cm at widest point. Cat-eye in shape. Large fibrous purulent mass present in wound bed centre, approximately the size of a large coin. Slight purulent odour noted. No other discharge evident. Wound bed mildly inflamed. Wound edges slightly raised. Peri wound skin red and inflamed to approximately 1 cm.
>
> Pt asked how long mass had been present. Pt reported mass present since shortly after wound separation. Pt asked if experiencing pain. Pt denied pain. Consent obtained to examine wound further. Mass palpated and gently removed. No bleeding or further discharge noted. Wound bed underneath is reddened.

This example demonstrates:

- a clear sequence
- factual, observable language
- inclusion of patient input and consent
- documentation of what occurred during examination

No diagnosis is made. No interpretation is imposed. This entry goes a little further than most examinations in that it mentions the mass was removed during the process. This is an example of a what I call a Disruptive Care Event. For more information about these events, please refer to chapter five.

Example: examination using touch

> O/E:
> Scabbed wound noted on right forearm. Surrounding skin inflamed. Scab mobile on palpation. Purulent discharge noted beneath scab.

This brief entry records:

- what was felt
- what was observed

It doesn't explain why it mattered. That comes later.

Example: examination using hearing

> Pt sitting upright on stretcher. Increased respiratory rate. Laboured breathing. Minimal audible airflow. Pt alert and oriented. No pain reported. Mood anxious.

Here, the absence of sound is an observation, not a conclusion. It allows the seriousness of the situation to be recognised without overstatement.

Example: examination using smell

> O/E:
> IDC in situ, patent and draining. Urinary bag contains approximately 100 mL white, purulent, foul-smelling discharge. Surrounding skin intact. No other signs or symptoms of infection noted at time of examination.

Here, the smell is recorded as an objective finding. The documentation remains factual and restrained.

A Key Point

During examination, your documentation should answer one question:

"What did I find?"

Not:

- What do I think it means?
- What should happen next?

Those elements belong to later stages of care and documentation.

Clear, descriptive examination notes demonstrate clinical competence, support safe decision-making, and provide a solid foundation for whatever follows.

Chapter 4: The Specific Nursing Task

All nursing care involves intervention at most and interaction at least. As a nurse, you are either helping a patient do something they can do but are struggling with, or you are doing something for them that they cannot do for themselves. This foundational level of care is made up of a series of actions that, when taken together, achieve the required outcome. These principles apply across the broad spectrum of nursing interventions.

Some aspects of care can be recorded in general terms. Others require more detailed documentation. Generally, the interventions that need to be recorded in greater detail are those that are medically based or procedural in nature. A useful guide is this: if you are required to complete a nursing competency to perform the task, you should document the process you followed to complete it.

A Quick Note About Competency and Scope of Practice

After you graduate from your nursing course, you should have all the basic skills needed to practice your level of nursing safely. However, it is important to know that there are some additional skills you need to develop related specifically to the nursing area you work in. Often, these are more technical procedures, such as catheterisation, specialised wound care or Advanced Life Support. These additional skills are learnt at your workplace, or you may need to attend a specialised training session to acquire them. Referred to as competencies, they are a bit like the merit badges awarded to scouts. The scout demonstrates skill in a certain area and is awarded a badge. A nurse acquires a new skill and gains a competency.

The sum of your basic nursing skills and your additional competencies in your field of nursing are referred to collectively as your Scope of Practice. Because nursing interventions can have the capacity to harm as well as heal, it is essential that you only perform those advanced nursing interventions that you have achieved a competency in. Acting outside your Scope of Practice is dangerous to the patient and to you professionally. Do not operate outside your Scope of Practice! If you are asked to do something and

> **you do not have the competency to perform it, tell the person making the request that you cannot do that task as you haven't been trained in it and help find a way for someone else who has the competency to perform that task. Seek to increase your Scope of Practice as much as possible. It will broaden your understanding of nursing, increase your care capacity and make you very much more employable.**

There are two main reasons for documenting a clinical procedure step by step. The first is that it creates a clear record of what was done to the patient. This is invaluable for ongoing care and essential if a clinical review is ever required. In this way, documentation protects both the patient and the nurse.

The second reason is educational. Writing out the procedure you followed reinforces it. In effect, you perform the task once clinically and then repeat it cognitively through documentation. This doubles your learning and provides an opportunity to reflect on your practice. Reflecting on your practice, particularly when your process is captured in your clinical notes, improves your nursing.

As a student nurse on placement with a Hospital in the Home service, I was once asked to administer a Clexane injection. I had given similar injections before and did not anticipate any issues. However, when I inserted the needle and began depressing the plunger, the patient cried out in pain and described the sensation as burning. I felt terrible — I had never had a patient react that way before.

After returning to the hospital, as part of my documentation, I reflected on what happened. As a result, I decided to research techniques for reducing patient discomfort during subcutaneous injections. I found an approach that I believed would help and practised it deliberately. It involved taking a firm pinch of the patient's abdominal tissue, so the sensation of pressure was prominent, then slowly and evenly depressing the plunger while gradually releasing that pressure to allow the medication to disperse subcutaneously. At a later visit, the supervising nurse asked a patient who gave the best injections, and she pointed to me. Reflective practice enabled me to keep my patients more comfortable and improved my quality of care.

As an aside, it has been many years since I last administered Clexane, and current best practice should always be consulted. The point of this example is not the technique itself, and this should not be read as current clinical instruction. Clinical techniques and best practice change over time. The purpose of the example is to show how reflection on practice can lead to improved nursing care.

Whenever you perform an intervention, you should also check that it has achieved its intended effect — even when the intervention is observational. During the night shifts I completed as a trainee nurse, I checked my patients hourly. Rather than simply noting that a patient was in bed,

I would observe one full breathing cycle and document that I had seen the patient breathing. Instead of writing “Pt sleeping”, I would write “Pt sleeping. Observed for one breath cycle.” This made it clear that the patient was alive and breathing at the time of review, rather than simply assumed to be so.

During clinical procedures, it is also important to document details about any devices used if they are relevant to ongoing care or review. For example, when recording a catheter change, noting the catheter size reinforces correct equipment selection and provides clarity if the record is later reviewed. While device details are often included in medical orders, documenting them confirms that you checked and followed those orders.

It is also good practice to confirm that a device is functioning correctly and to document that you observed it working. This communicates to the next nurse that the device was operating as intended at the conclusion of your care and provides assurance during any subsequent review.

Patient Consent

One aspect of care that should always be documented when performing a clinical procedure is patient consent. This is important not only from a clinical and legal perspective, but also because it reinforces to the patient that you are mindful of what you are asking them to undergo.

I recall working as a community nurse administering intravenous antibiotics to a patient. When the time came to give the medication, I asked the patient for her consent. She looked at me and said that I was the only nurse who had ever asked her for consent and asked why. I explained, as politely as possible, that she was trusting me to introduce a chemical substance into her body, and that the least I could do was ask her permission. She greatly appreciated that perspective and I was glad that something so simple increased patient trust and comfort.

Documenting This

The following examples are documentation examples only. They are not procedural instructions. Any clinical intervention must be performed only where clinically appropriate, within the nurse's scope of practice, and in accordance with current local policy, training, and competency requirements.

Documenting the steps you took during a clinical procedure is essential to safe and effective patient care. Your documentation should be clear, concise, factual, and free of unnecessary detail or descriptive language. Each statement should describe exactly what occurred.

One way to think about documenting a procedure is to compare it to a function in computer programming. A function is a series of instructions that, when carried out correctly, return a desired result. Documenting a nursing procedure follows the same principle: you record each step taken, and the "return value" is the successful completion of the task.

When reading the nursing encounters below, you will notice some abbreviations. It is your responsibility to ensure that you only use approved abbreviations when documenting patient care. Some abbreviations used here may no longer be accepted, as standards change over time. Most local health services have a policy containing a list of approved abbreviations. Grab a copy and learn them.

As mentioned previously, how you write your notes reflects your thinking, which in turn reflects how you approach your clinical practice and patient care. When documenting a nursing intervention, I often began this section of my notes with the heading:

Procedure:

What followed was a record of the steps taken during the procedure only. I did not repeat information already documented elsewhere, such as how the patient was found or what was identified on examination. The examples below are provided to illustrate how to document procedures, not to teach the procedures themselves. Ideally, your documentation should always align with established local health policy and procedure.

Example: basic wound care

> Procedure:
> Sterile field established.
> PPE applied and verbal consent obtained.
> Wound washed with N/S using ANTT. Some slough removed and discarded.
> Betadine applied to wound bed.
> Zetuvit 10x10 applied.
> Secured with Mefix.

This entry records the establishment of a sterile field, use of PPE, and confirmation of consent. It documents cleaning the wound using Aseptic Non-Touch Technique (ANTT), removal of slough, application of antiseptic, and dressing selection. Including the dressing size assists the next nurse in preparing appropriate supplies. When I was nursing, N/S was an accepted abbreviation of normal saline.

Example: IV antibiotic administration

> Procedure:
> Medication order checked and in date. IVAB prepared as per policy.
> New IV bag label applied.
> IV antibiotic order double-checked with RN Smith.
> Pt verbally identified.
> Pt verbal consent obtained.
> PPE applied.
> Previous IV bag and line removed and inspected — no kinks or blockages noted.
>
> Line inserted, primed, and checked — no air, leaks, or blockages observed. IV antibiotics set up via infusion pump.
> Cannula swabbed with antiseptic.
> Line connected to cannula.
> Infusion set to 125 mL/hr as per order.
> Infusion observed — pump functioning normally.
> IV line secured for patient comfort.

This documentation confirms medication safety checks, patient identification, aseptic preparation, equipment integrity, correct infusion rate, and the IV line being secured.

Example: indwelling catheter change

Procedure:
Medical order checked and in date.
Patient verbal consent obtained.
Previous catheter balloon deflated (8 mL in balloon).
Previous catheter and leg bag removed. 800 mL clear straw-coloured urine in bag.
Gloves removed and hand hygiene performed.
Sterile field established using catheter pack.
Double sterile gloves applied.
Area cleansed with N/S.
Outer gloves removed.
Catheter balloon checked — no defects noted.
Lubricant applied via catheter-tipped syringe.
16 Fr catheter inserted using sterile technique as per order.
Urine free-flowing; catheter patent and draining straw coloured clear urine.
Balloon inflated with 10 mL sterile water.
Positioning checked.
Leg bag attached.
Catheter and leg bag secured to patient's right leg as per patient preference.

This entry demonstrates order verification, consent, removal of previous equipment, establishment of a sterile field, correct insertion technique, confirmation of catheter function, and securing for patient comfort.

A Time Saver with a Warning

Nurses have limited time to complete detailed documentation. One time-saving strategy I used was to keep templates for common procedures on my computer. When it came time to write my notes, I would copy and paste the relevant template into the clinical record. This method also provided a regular reminder for correct procedure, ensuring both my practice and my notes aligned with organisational policy and best practice.

However, I strongly caution against blindly copying and pasting notes. A diligent nurse will read through the pasted content as if it were a new entry, ensuring that every detail accurately reflects the care provided.

These examples are not exhaustive and are not intended to teach procedural technique. They are provided solely to demonstrate how to document the specific nursing task you performed in a way that is clear, defensible, and useful to those who continue the patient's care.

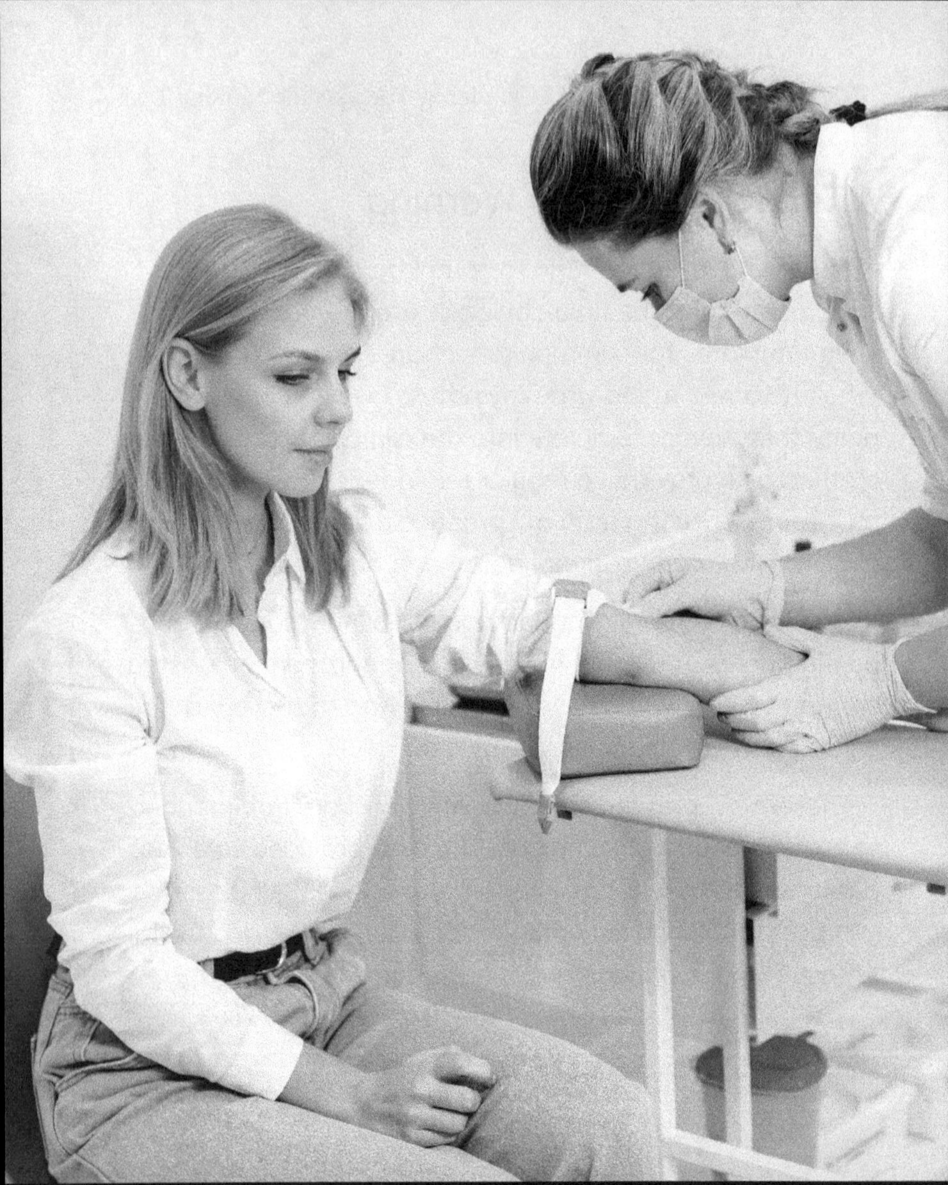

Take every opportunity to widen your scope of practice! Make it a habit to record your Professional Development courses, dates and what you learned.

It is invaluable!

Chapter 5: Disruptive Care Events

The previous chapter described the clinical processes that occur as part of routine patient care, following an expected clinical pathway. Most catheter changes, wound dressings, and IV antibiotic administrations occur without incident. However, sometimes things happen.

A **disruptive care event** is any occurrence during care that alters, interrupts, or complicates the expected process. This does not always involve an immediate medical emergency, although it certainly can. A disruptive care event may be additional information provided by the patient or family, an unexpected response to treatment, behaviour that impacts staff safety, or a situation that requires escalation or alteration of care.

When such an event occurs, it must be managed within the context of holistic nursing practice. Use your clinical judgement to determine whether the issue can safely wait until the specific nursing task is completed, or whether it must be addressed immediately.

As part of your nursing role, you should remain alert to the possibility of disruptive care events. Awareness allows a degree of preparation and reduces the likelihood of being caught off guard. At the same time, it is important to remain present and focused on the care you are providing. Do not become so preoccupied with anticipating problems that you overburden yourself. Be aware, but not hyper vigilant — particularly as most anticipated issues never eventuate.

Chaperoning: A Common and Preventable Risk

A common consideration to avoid a disruptive care event is the need for a chaperone.

While working as a community nurse, I once cared for a 19-year-old female patient who required dressing of a sacral pilonidal sinus. At the time, I was a male nurse in my forties. After commencing the encounter and noting that the patient was alone, I offered a chaperone and explained that this would protect both her and me. She agreed.

I asked a female receptionist at the community clinic to act as a chaperone. She stood at the back of the room during the procedure. The dressing was completed without incident, and the consent for and presence of the chaperone were documented.

A Cautionary Tale

A chaperone should always be offered when providing care to a patient of the opposite sex, regardless of circumstances, and the patient's response documented.

I once cared for a female patient who was older than me and herself a registered nurse. Something about the situation triggered my caution. I attempted to arrange for another clinician to provide care, but the patient insisted the dressing be done immediately. In the difficulty of the moment, I failed to offer a chaperone.

Appropriate nursing care was provided and documented. Despite this, a complaint was later made. I share this experience to reinforce a simple principle: **good nursing care and clear documentation protect you as much as they protect the patient**.

Additional Information That Alters Care

Disruptive care events may involve information that emerges during care and alters how that care should proceed.

On one visit, I was dressing a patient's wounds at home following hospital discharge. I noted full ashtrays and a strong smell of tobacco. The patient had also been provided with an oxygen concentrator. At the time, it was against NSW Health policy for oxygen concentrators to be loaned to active smokers due to fire risk.

The patient was not smoking during the visit but was wearing nasal prongs connected to the concentrator. I warned him of the dangers of smoking while using oxygen and explained the fire risk. He appeared indifferent. The education and his response were documented.

Weeks later, the patient sustained a burn while smoking and required hospitalisation. My documentation confirmed that he had been warned on two occasions. This information was critical in reviewing the incident.

Unexpected Patient Practices

Another example involved an elderly patient with a foot wound. His daughter informed me that he removed his dressings after visits and scrubbed the wound with brandy using a clean flannel. I advised her to encourage adherence to the prescribed care plan.

On review, the wound bed was exceptionally healthy, with excellent granulation tissue and no signs of infection. While I continued to dress the wound as per protocol, the experience informed my future practice — particularly around thorough wound cleansing in patients with reduced sensation.

Difficult and Distressing Encounters

Some disruptive care events negatively impact staff safety or emotional wellbeing and must be addressed promptly and documented.

In one experience, a colleague reported being photographed by a patient during wound care and how uncomfortable it made her feel. When the same patient attempted to photograph me, I clearly stated that I did not consent and would leave and escalate if he continued. He complied, and the incident did not happen again. I made sure my documentation recorded his actions and my response. The next time my colleague dressed this patient's wounds, she made sure to tell the patient that he did not have her consent to photograph her. There were no further attempts by the patient to photograph staff from that point on.

Emotional and Psychological Care

Not all nursing care is physical.

During a palliative care admission, I asked a patient how she was feeling. She replied sharply, "What do you think?" I reflected briefly and responded that if I were in her position, I would be frightened. She admitted that she was terrified.

I asked her if she was religious and she said she was. We talked about her life of devotion, and that God loves His children. These aspects were discussed in very general terms, without specific religious doctrine. Through that conversation, grounded in her faith, the patient became calmer and more at peace. The essence of the discussion and its impact on her wellbeing were documented. It should be noted that I did not espouse any particular view.

I provided an opportunity for the patient to reflect on her own beliefs and find comfort in them. When patients are not religious, similar conversations can focus on meaning, achievements, and valued relationships.

Challenging Behaviour and Boundaries

Some patients express frustration through difficult behaviour. I once cared for a patient who demanded higher doses of opioid analgesia than prescribed and threatened discharge against medical advice. I explained that nurses are legally not allowed to increase medication doses and explained the implications of discharge against medical advice clearly. When he realised that discharge would remove him from the procedure queue, he chose to stay. The interaction was documented in detail to inform ongoing care and staff awareness.

Disruptive Care Events During Specific Nursing Tasks

Disruptive care events may also occur **during** a nursing procedure. When this happens, they should be documented as part of the task itself to preserve chronology and clarity.

Examples include allergic reactions during IV antibiotic administration, unexpected bleeding during wound care, or acute deterioration during routine observations.

Documenting This

Disruptive care events can be documented in three main ways:

1. **Before the specific nursing task**, when the event informs how care proceeds
2. **After the task**, when the event is incidental but relevant
3. **During the task**, when the event directly alters or interrupts care

The clinical notes below are written to document the examples provided in this chapter. They demonstrate how these situations can be recorded clearly and defensibly.

Example: chaperone offered prior to care

> For pilonidal sinus dressing:
> Pt offered chaperone. Accepted.
> Chaperone: receptionist Silvia Smith.
> Present by consent at back of room.
> O/E:
> Wound located ...

This entry records the offer and acceptance of a chaperone, identifies who the chaperone was, and documents their position in the room.

Example: discharge against medical advice discussion

> Called to pt's room. Pt expressed frustration at RNs not giving him a higher opioid analgesia dose and expressed a desire to self-discharge.
> Pt informed that discharge would be against medical advice.
> Pt informed that nurses may legally only administer opioid analgesia as charted by MO.
> Pt expressed dissatisfaction and reaffirmed discharge against medical advice. Pt requested that, post discharge, RN notify him when it was his time for his procedure.
> Pt informed that discharge would remove him from procedure queue.
> Pt declined discharge. Pt unhappy but settled.

This entry notes the patient's frustration and the reasons for it. It notes that the patient was provided with education about the legal framework surrounding opioid medication administration. It records his response and his expressed wishes for discharge against medical advice. It notes that the patient was informed of the consequences of his choice and his decision to not proceed. Lastly, it records his mood at the close of the encounter.

Example: disruptive event during wound care

> For wound care.
>
> Previous dressings removed. Some strike-through noted.
>
> O/E:
>
> Wound to left knee approx. 6 cm × 5 cm.
>
> Granulating tissue. Some slough. No signs of infection.
>
> Upper thigh markedly bruised.
>
> Pt's wife reports recent fall.
>
> Procedure:
>
> Wound washed with N/S using ANTT.
>
> Black exudate noted from 2 mm opening. Applied pressure. Ineffective.
>
> Options explained. Pt opted for exploration.
>
> Large volume black exudate and congealed blood expressed.
>
> Wound cleansed and dressed with Zetuvit 10 × 10.
>
> Mefix applied.
>
> Pt and wife educated re signs and symptoms of infection and advised to seek GP or ED review if unwell. Pt and his wife agreed to do so.

This example notes the care process and the deviation caused by the disruptive care event, which was a large amount of black congealed fluid being expressed from the wound. It notes that options were offered and what the patient chose to do. It also notes that the patient and his wife received education relating to signs and symptoms of infection and what to do should they occur. It recorded that they understood what was required of them. In this real-life example, the education proved to be essential as two days later, the patient experienced symptoms of infection, and presented to a healthcare facility where he was prescribed antibiotics.

Example: incidental disruptive event documented after care (smoking with oxygen therapy)

> Pt warned of dangers of smoking with O_2 concentrator.
> Pt appeared ambivalent.

This brief entry documents education provided and the patient's response.

Example: additional information provided by family

> RN informed by pt's daughter that pt removes dressings post-visit and cleans wound using brandy and flannel.
> Pt and carer advised of potential for delayed healing if treatment plan not followed.
> Pt's daughter aware but willing to allow pt to continue as he chooses.

This entry notes the alteration to wound care, the advice given against altering accepted treatment and the carer's response.

Example: anaphylaxis during IV antibiotic administration

For IVABs.

O/E:

16 Fr Cannula in pt's right Cub Foss. Pt's cannula site has no signs or symptoms of infection.

Procedure:

Obs as charted.

Cannula cleaned. Flushed with 10 mL N/S. Patent.

IVAB's checked with RN Green against medication order.

Line inserted into bag and primed. No air bubbles, kinks, particles or blockages.

IVAB's administered.

Pt admitted to Community Health.

During the admission, pt became agitated. Called out 'Itch! Itch!'

Infusion stopped.

O/E:

Pt developed hives on arms and legs. Airway still patent. No stridor. Pt breathing normally. Alert and oriented. No pain. Mood is panicked. Sitting upright in wheelchair.

(Continued next page)

1135	Anaphylaxis protocol initiated. Pt given IM 0.5 mg adrenaline as per protocol outer right mid-thigh. Obs as charted. Within acceptable parameters. Help sought from RACF staff. Advised that a doctor will be there this afternoon. Returned to pt.
1136	Obs as charted. Within acceptable parameters. Ambulance called.
1137	Obs as charted. Within acceptable parameters.
1138	Obs as charted. Within acceptable parameters.
1139	Obs as charted. Within acceptable parameters.
1140	O/E: pt still has hives. Airway still patent. No stridor. Pt breathing normal. Alert and oriented. No pain. Mood is panicked. Sitting upright in wheelchair. Pt given IM 0.5 mg adrenaline as per protocol outer left mid-thigh. Obs as charted. Within acceptable parameters.
1141	Obs as charted. Within acceptable parameters.
1142	Obs as charted. Within acceptable parameters.

I'll stop here, but this cycle would continue as per the Anaphylaxis Protocol until the ambulance arrived. When the ambulance arrived, the entry would be something like this:

1150	Paramedics arrived. Pt handed over and in paramedic care.

At this point, the nursing responsibility ends. Care provided by others is not documented in your clinical notes.

This entry follows the specific nursing task, then goes straight into the disruptive care event, specifically recording the time that nursing interventions occurred and what those interventions were. This is extremely important and highlights the need for nurses to be able to record information on the fly if they do not have access to the patient's clinical record at the time the disruption occurred.

Example: patient self-removes PICC line.

This example refers to me as a patient when I was hospitalised for a Subarachnoid Haemorrhage late 2022. Although I have no memory of the event, my dear wife related to me that I pulled the inserted PICC line out of my arm at some point during my care. If I was the nurse writing up this event, I would write something like this:

> O/E:
>
> Pt has self-removed PICC line. Some bleeding. No signs or symptoms of infection. Pt resting but rousable. Normal breathing. No pain. Mood is agitated. Pt able to move but not able to self-care.
>
> Procedure:
>
> Direct pressure applied to stop bleeding.
>
> Washed with N/S.
>
> Adhesive NAD applied.
>
> NIC informed of self-removal.

Notice here that a quick assessment of the patient was also recorded. As I don't remember the incident, I do not know how much blood was lost when I self-removed the PICC line. A quick examination lets me know - and the record reflect - that an assessment was performed and that the patient was stable, even though stemming the blood and washing and dressing the wound are routine. I also documented that I escalated the problem to the Nurse in Charge so that alternative IV medication administration could be attended to.

Key Message

Routine care does not always proceed as planned. When it does not, assess the situation, act according to policy and professional judgement, and document clearly. Good documentation ensures continuity of care, protects staff, and supports the best possible outcomes for patients.

Chapter 6: Concluding the Patient Encounter

> Pt happy with service. No complaints voiced.

Concluding a patient encounter is just as important as every other aspect of nursing care. It is not simply a matter of finishing a task and moving on. A well-concluded encounter serves two important functions.

Firstly, it ensures that the patient understands what has happened, what is required of them, and what will occur next in their care. Knowing the pathway forward reduces uncertainty and anxiety. Many patient concerns can be eased simply by explaining what comes next and what the patient should expect. This is particularly important for patients who must suddenly prepare themselves for treatment or investigation.

As a student nurse on placement in a private orthopaedic ward, I often saw patients asked to stop eating breakfast or washing because they were scheduled for post-operative X-rays and needed to leave immediately. This frequently occurred the day after surgery, when patients were tired, sore, hungry, and vulnerable. Clear explanation and reassurance in these moments can make a significant difference to how the patient experiences their care.

Secondly, concluding the encounter well leaves the patient with a positive impression. It reinforces confidence in the treatment provided and in the healthcare system more broadly. This is especially important for anxious or nervous patients, who may otherwise become distressed or resistant to care.

Patient Education at the End of the Encounter

Concluding the patient encounter often begins with education related to ongoing or future care. Nurses sometimes think of education only in terms of explaining medical conditions or terminology. In this context, patient education refers to anything the patient needs to know moving forward.

This may include:

- What to look out for
- How to care for themselves
- When and where the next appointment will be
- What to do if a problem arises

Any education provided should be documented.

As a community nurse, I often concluded clinic visits by making the patient's next appointment. This involved reviewing their wound or catheter care schedule, booking the appointment in the system, and providing the patient with a reminder card. I would then ensure the patient had all their belongings and walk them to the door. Before concluding the visit, I would take a moment to observe how the patient appeared in response to the care provided, as this is also important to document.

When No Education Is Required

Not all patient encounters conclude with formal education. Sometimes the task is completed, the patient is settled, and the nurse moves on to the next responsibility. In these situations, it is still important to document the patient's response to care.

Patient satisfaction — or dissatisfaction — is a meaningful indicator. Patients are inherently vulnerable, and vulnerable people often respond emotionally rather than logically. Patients are unlikely to remember precise blood test results or imaging findings. What they will remember is whether they were treated with kindness, respect, and dignity.

I recall an encounter where a patient called my student nurse and me into her room in an agitated tone. She complained that a physiotherapist had been too rough with her earlier that day. I knew the physiotherapist to be competent and professional, but that was not the point.

After listening to the patient, I told her I would speak to the physiotherapist. She was satisfied with this response.

I did speak to the physiotherapist and suggested that an apology might help. Later that day, the patient called us back into her room to thank us. The physiotherapist had apologised, and the patient felt heard.

This example highlights an important truth: patients will often forgive system failures, delays, or even mistakes. What they struggle to tolerate is feeling dismissed or treated unkindly.

Documenting This

When documenting the conclusion of a patient encounter, record what education was provided (if any), the patient's response, and whether any concerns were raised.

Example: wound care clinic appointment

If a patient attended the clinic for wound care for the first time, and education was provided, documentation might look like this:

> Pt educated re signs and symptoms of infection and what to do if they occur.
> Pt acknowledged understanding.
> Next appointment made. Pt aware and given reminder card.
> No other issues expressed.
>
> Pt happy with service. No complaints voiced.

Example: new patient orientation re toilet

If a patient on the ward self-mobilised to the toilet and that patient was new to the hospital experience, you might write something along the lines of:

> Pt expressed need to toilet. Pt educated re toilet call bells and what to do. Pt self-mobilised to toilet. Reports PUIT. No incidents. Returned to bed.

When I was nursing, PUIT was an acceptable shorthand for "passed urine in toilet".

If no education was required and there were no outstanding issues, documentation may simply state:

> Pt happy with service. No complaints voiced.

If concerns were raised, these should be documented along with how they will be addressed. For example:

> Pt frustrated with physiotherapy session this AM.
> Offered to speak to physio regarding concerns.
> Pt agreeable to this plan.
> No other issues identified.

Alternatively, I write:

> No issues identified or noted.

Any agreed-upon actions should then be recorded in the Plan section of the notes. Documenting the plan for continued care is the focus of the next chapter.

Chapter 7: Planning Future Care

A Simple Story

Earlier, I mentioned an ex-US Navy nurse tutor I had at university who taught me that if air is going in and out and blood is going 'round and 'round, it is not a medical emergency. This same nurse, always full of practical teaching moments, taught me another important lesson.

She told us about an occasion when a loved one of hers was in hospital while she was not present. Frustrated by what appeared to be a lack of obvious care, she went to the hospital to be with them. It wasn't long before the nurse allocated to her loved one entered the room to perform routine care. When the moment was appropriate, my tutor asked the nurse a very simple question:

"What's the plan?"

The nurse had no idea what she meant.

A discussion followed, during which my tutor explained that there should be a plan in place for her loved one's care - and for every patient. Experience has taught me that not only should such a plan exist, but the nurse providing care should be aware of it and understand their role in carrying it out.

Patients and their families draw great comfort from nurses who can explain what is happening, what is planned, and where the patient is in relation to their treatment pathway. There is often an assumption that doctors will explain this. While many Medical Officers are excellent communicators, my experience is that communication often falls to nurses, whether intentionally or not.

This is not a criticism of doctors. I have worked with many highly skilled and compassionate physicians. However, I cannot guarantee that every patient will receive clear explanations from a Medical Officer. What I can say is that patients consistently turn to nurses for clarity, reassurance, and guidance.

Thinking Ahead as Part of Nursing Care

Unless you are documenting a patient's discharge, every time you record a specific nursing task you should also be thinking about what comes next. Planning future care helps keep the patient on an established clinical pathway and reinforces continuity of care.

This plan:

- Keeps future care clear in your own mind
- Helps other nurses provide consistent care
- Reassures patients and their families

- Reduces the likelihood of missed tasks

Importantly, this is not the full nursing care plan or a formal clinical pathway. It is a short-term, practical reflection of what needs to happen next in relation to the care you provide.

Your plan should include:

- Specific nursing tasks you intend to perform, such as medication administration and patient observations
- Outstanding routine personal care, such as showers, toilet, etc
- Medical orders that need to be followed up

Documenting This

When documenting future care, I begin with a simple heading:

Plan:

Under this heading, I list the tasks that need to be completed. My nursing notes throughout the shift should reflect that I am working through this list. If a task cannot be completed, it must be handed over to the next nurse.

Example: ward patient

Imagine you are caring for a patient on a medical-surgical ward during a 7:00 am shift. On reviewing the notes and handover, you note that:

- Blood tests have been ordered
- Daily weighing is required

Your plan might look like this:

Plan:
BD obs
Meds as charted
For routine personal care.
Daily AM weight pre-breakfast
Organise pathology

In this example:

- BD (bis die) means twice daily (many services now prefer “twice daily” written in full)
- Meds as charted indicates medications will be administered as per the medication chart
- Routine personal care refers to hygiene and washing
- Daily AM weight pre-breakfast ensures consistency of when patient weighs are conducted.
- Organise pathology reminds you to ensure blood collection occurs

Again, follow your local policy regarding abbreviations.

Example: community wound care

In community nursing, dressing frequency is often determined by clinical judgement. If I felt a patient required a wound review, my plan might read:

> Plan:
> For wound care Tuesdays and Fridays
> Organise wound review with GP

This records both the ongoing care and the need for review. As part of your responsibility, it is important to follow up on these plans where possible. If a task cannot be completed, it must be handed over clearly.

Where the Plan Sits in Care

Establishing a forward care plan completes the documentation cycle for a specific nursing task. It ties together what was done, what was identified, and what needs to happen next.

However, not everything a nurse does fits neatly into a task or plan. Many actions occur alongside care—phone calls, arrangements, requests, and small supportive actions. These actions are incidental to care, but still important.

Documenting incidental nursing care is the focus of the next chapter.

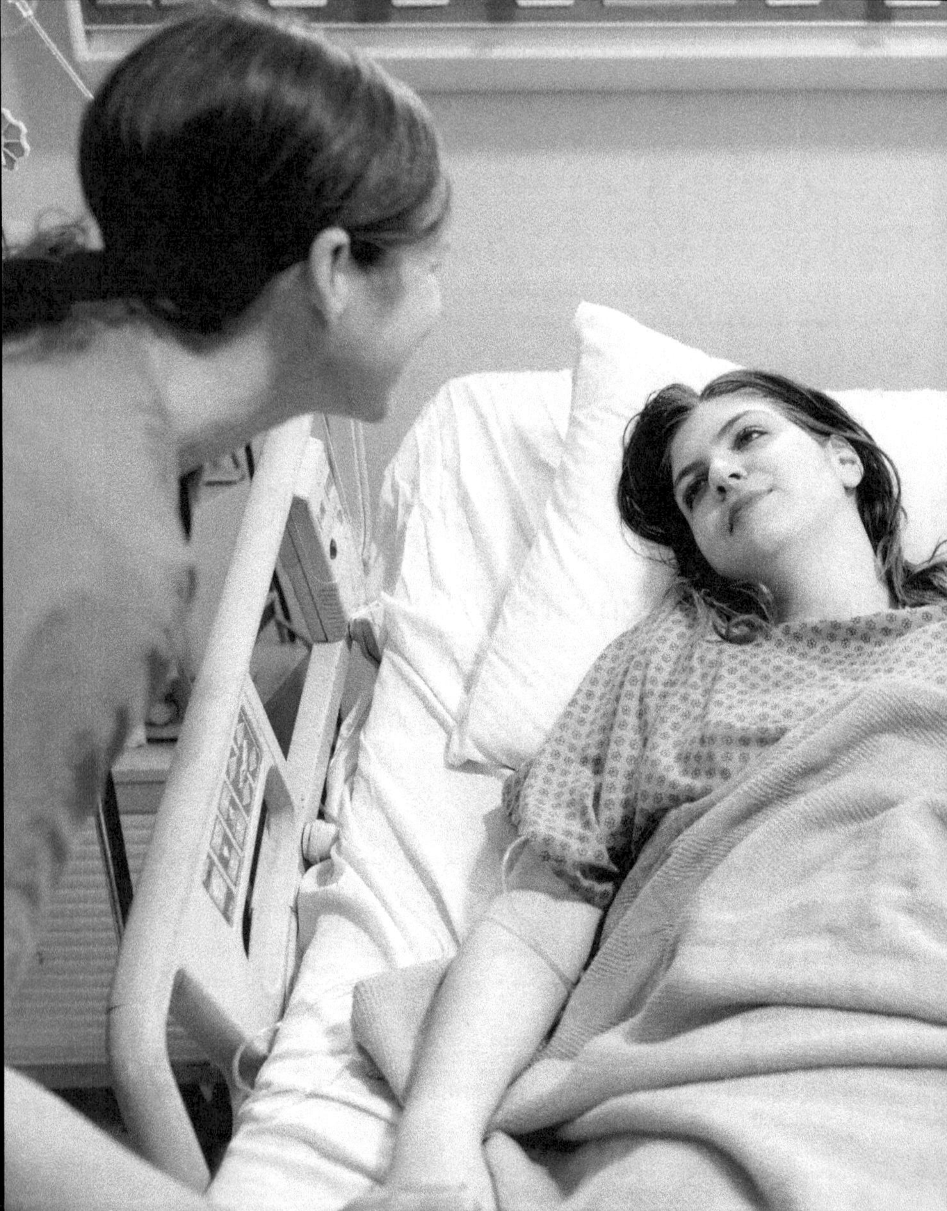

It is not your job to save a patient's life. It is your job to do your job well. Even the most skilled nurses have lost patients.

Chapter 8: Incidental Nursing Care

Not all nursing involves therapeutic procedures. Often, it is the simple, mundane tasks that make up a substantial proportion of nursing care. These tasks act like mortar between the bricks of specific nursing interventions, holding the patient's overall nursing care plan together. Incidental nursing care is often integrated into routine care, but its importance cannot be overstated. Among other things, it enables the nursing care plan to proceed as smoothly as possible, leading to positive nursing experiences and outcomes.

What Is Incidental Nursing Care?

Incidental nursing care is any care that happens alongside, around, or because of therapeutic nursing tasks but is not the primary clinical intervention. Often, it is routine, brief, and practical — but it is still nursing care.

One good example, covered in greater depth later in this chapter, is nursing care collaboration. It has often been said that much of patient care planning occurs in ward corridors, when nurses encounter one another during routine tasks and discuss patient care as they go. These impromptu conversations frequently lead to coordinated care initiatives that directly benefit patients.

Incidental nursing care usually occurs around specific nursing tasks, though it can also occur during one. For example, I was present during a medical emergency in a High Dependency Unit when the patient rolled over and vomited onto the bed and floor. In addition to managing the medical emergency, we now also had to address a workplace hazard involving clinical waste. While the immediate medical care continued, I asked a nurse who was standing by without a defined role to take over from me, which she did. I then went to the linen cupboard, collected towels, and returned to the bedside. Working around the clinical team, I cleaned the vomit and removed the hazard, allowing medical care to continue with reduced risk.

Although cleaning vomit was incidental to the emergency care being provided, incidental does not mean unimportant. In fact, incidental care often has the greatest impact on patient comfort, dignity, and trust.

Why Incidental Care Must Be Documented

Incidental nursing care must be documented because it provides a complete picture of patient care and the role of staff in delivering that care. Documenting incidental nursing care demonstrates — and records — holistic nursing practice. It also protects the nurse and the health service by showing that patient needs were identified, reasonable efforts were made to assist the patient, and the patient's response to care was noted.

This documentation clarifies the level of support a patient required at a particular point in time and helps prevent under-documentation of nursing workload; an important consideration when determining staffing needs. It also assists other nurses to understand patient mobility, independence, activity tolerance, and any changing care requirements. Incidental nursing care occurs as a routine part of treatment and should be noted accordingly.

Documenting This

The examples below do not cover every possible situation. Instead, they draw on real-life experiences to demonstrate how incidental nursing care may be documented. Some incidental tasks are routine and can be recorded in a brief, general manner. Others require more detailed documentation because of their complexity or significance.

As with specific nursing tasks, it is up to you to determine how much detail is required. The guiding principle remains the same: keep sentences brief, factual, and detailed enough to give another nurse or a clinical reviewer a clear picture of what happened.

As a small aside, when documenting incidental nursing care, I often recorded the time the event occurred. While this is not always necessary — particularly in electronic records that are time-stamped — there can be a discrepancy between when an event occurs and when it is documented.

Some forms of incidental nursing care include:

- Routine personal care
- Toileting and mobility assistance
- Assisting with therapeutic measures
- Supporting diagnostic and treatment processes
- Escalating patient care
- Communication and coordination of care
- Emotional, social, and supportive care

The sections below provide examples of how these forms of incidental care may arise and how they can be documented.

As mentioned earlier, incidental nursing care is often recorded as a simple statement or a few short sentences. For example, if I were escorting a patient to imaging — a common occurrence in Emergency — I might document it as follows:

1335	Pt escorted to imaging.
1350	Pt RTW cubicle 16. All monitoring equipment reattached. Pt resting in bed. Plan: Routine obs.

RTW was an accepted abbreviation for "Returned to Ward". This entry records the escort, the patient's return location, reconnection of monitoring equipment, the patient's condition, and the forward plan.

Escalation of Patient Care

Another example of incidental nursing care is patient escalation. If I felt the need to escalate a patient following routine observations, I might record something like this:

1137	Obs as charted. HR 110 bpm at rest. RR elevated at 18 bpm. All other obs within acceptable parameters. No pain. Mood agitated. No nausea. No diaphoresis. No observable cause for increased HR. Able to reposition in bed. Escalated to NIC for immediate review. Plan: Follow up NIC review. Obs every 10 minutes until review.

This note highlights abnormal observations, documents further assessment, and records escalation to the Nurse in Charge (NIC). It also outlines a clear plan for ongoing monitoring and following up with the NIC, who has their own workload and is not simply waiting to be approached. It records the escalation and demonstrates appropriate judgement and follow up.

If no concerns were identified after the obs were taken, I would document it more simply:

1137	Obs as charted. Within acceptable parameters.

In my experience, many nurses I worked with wrote 'obs' or 'obs as charted', to record that the patient's observations were taken. While this may be generally accepted, it does not record a clinical judgement of those observations. For example, in my graduate year, a nurse tutor related a story in which he observed a new nurse in theatre, who was dutifully taking observations at set intervals of a patient in recovery. While this action was commendable, it fell short because although the new nurse was dutifully taking the patient's observations, she failed to notice that the patient's vital signs were deteriorating. Thankfully, a more senior nurse saw the patient, checked the observations, realised what was happening and took immediate action. By recording 'within acceptable parameters', if the observations are stable, a clinical judgement is attached to the observations themselves. This demonstrates that not only did the nurse take the observations but interpreted what they meant and acted accordingly.

Routine Personal Care

Routine personal care involves patient hygiene needs, including washing, showering, bed baths, oral care, shaving, and grooming. Ultimately, nurses aim to support patients to be as independent as possible with activities of daily living (ADLs), as independence is a good indicator of overall health.

That said, many patients require assistance. The level of assistance provided should be limited to what the patient cannot reasonably do themselves. Hospitals are not hotels, and part of nursing care involves encouraging independence where appropriate. As a new nurse, I once had a patient ring the call bell asking me to fluff her pillow. When I asked whether she could do it herself, she replied that she could. I gently reminded her that nursing care is focused on helping patients regain independence so they can return to everyday life.

When documenting routine personal care, the key focus is the level of assistance required, not merely the task. Changes in independence are clinically relevant and should be recorded. Routine care may also reveal skin integrity issues, mobility decline, pain, confusion, or fatigue.

For example, while assisting an older patient with washing, I noticed overlapping abdominal skin folds. When separated, the skin beneath was red, macerated, and broken down, revealing an unrecognised wound.

If documenting this today, I would write:

1035	Personal care attended to. Skin on pt's lower abdomen separated and washed. O/E: Wound to lower abdomen, hidden between skin folds. Skin red, raw, macerated. Light surface bleeding. Some odour present. No other signs of infection. Wound cleaned with N/S using ANTT. Macerated skin gently debrided with N/S-soaked gauze. Barrier cream applied. Large NAD placed between skin folds. Surrounding area dried. Pt dried, dressed, and returned to bed. Resting comfortably. Plan: Handover wound to nursing staff. Organise wound review and treatment plan.

If no issue had been identified, documentation would be much briefer:

1035	Personal care attended to. Pt dried, dressed, and returned to bed. Resting comfortably. No issues identified.

Toileting and Mobility Assistance

Toileting and mobility assistance includes helping patients with elimination needs and relocating for comfort or therapy. Documentation should note the assistance required, any aids used, and whether one or two staff were needed.

Toileting is a high-risk activity for falls. On my first ever paid shift as a nurse in HDU, a patient mobilised independently to the toilet. Shortly afterward, I heard a thud. I found the patient on the bathroom floor; he had fainted. The toilet bowl was filled with fresh blood. The patient was assisted back to bed and an immediate medical review initiated.

If documenting this today, I would write:

1445	Pt requested toilet. RN Khan advised pt could go. Pt self-mobilised.
1450	Pt found lying on toilet floor. RN Khan called to assist. O/E: Pt alert and oriented. Breathing normal. No pain. Mood anxious. B/O melena ++. Pt assisted to bed x2. Resting in bed. Plan: Immediate medical review. Immediate risk assessment. Inform NIC.

If no incident had occurred, today I would write something like the following:

1445	Pt self-mobilised to toilet.
1449	Pt self-mobilised to bed. Reports B/O. No issues raised.

When I was nursing B/O was an accepted abbreviation of 'bowels opened'. Melena is a medical term for blood in the stool. The ++ is a subjective record of the amount of blood noted. In this instance, '++' means that there was a lot of blood in the toilet! 'Assisted x2' or 'x2 assist' were accepted abbreviations for the number of nurses required to perform a task.

Therapeutic Measures

Nurses frequently perform simple therapeutic measures to assist patients. For example:

1643	2 L O_2 commenced via nasal prongs.

In the following example, cultural considerations arose during a routine ECG. Despite not being able to fully implement their request, the steps taken to accommodate them helped the patient and her husband feel more comfortable. If I was documenting this today, I would write something like:

1722	ECG ordered. Pt's husband requested female RN. Female RN unavailable. Situation explained. Consent obtained. ECG performed with pt kept covered. No complaints voiced. Results to MO Green.

If no issue arose, I would document as follows:

1722	ECG ordered. Consent obtained. Results to MO Green.

In these notes L refers to 'Litres' and O_2 was the accepted shorthand for oxygen. ECG is an accepted abbreviation for electrocardiogram. In other healthcare settings, it may be referred to as an EKG.

Emotional, Social, and Supportive Care

An essential component of nursing involves emotional, social, and supportive care. This includes listening, reassurance, advocacy, and recognising when ethical considerations outweigh routine processes.

For example, when I arrived for the morning shift at a rural hospital, I learned that a young patient had miscarried overnight. The pregnancy was less than a week from the gestational threshold that determined whether the loss would be managed as a stillbirth or as an early pregnancy loss. This distinction mattered, as it altered the processes that followed — including how the fetus was handled, what options were offered to the woman, and which support pathways were activated.

I asked the night shift nurses whether the woman had been offered the opportunity to see her baby. They told me that she had been offered this option, but at the time she declined. She simply wanted to leave.

I expressed my concern that decisions made in the immediate aftermath of such a loss may not always reflect what a patient ultimately wants. Grief can be overwhelming, and people often respond by trying to escape the situation as quickly as possible. I suggested that we contact the woman once more and offer her a final opportunity to see her baby, so that she could make that decision after having time to think. I also noted that, from a professional and ethical perspective, it is better to offer choice more than once than to deny it entirely. Should the decision ever be questioned, it is far more defensible to show that care was taken to ensure the woman was fully informed and supported, rather than relying solely on policy or an initial refusal.

Together, the nursing team agreed to contact the woman to confirm her wishes. Later in the shift, I learned that she had decided she did want to see her baby. The body was respectfully and gently wrapped in a clean towel, and a small flower was placed on the blanket beside it. The woman was given the opportunity to see her baby in a calm and dignified manner.

Although no additional clinical procedures were required, the nursing care in this situation involved advocacy and ensuring the patient had the opportunity to make an informed decision when she was able. The nursing care also required careful attention to policy, sensitivity in communication, and advocacy to ensure the woman understood her options. This type of care is often incidental to routine nursing tasks, but it is no less important. This experience occurred while I was still within my graduate nursing year. Even as a very new nurse, it reinforced for me that advocating for patients is not dependent on seniority.

If I were recording this today, I would write something like this:

0730	D/W night staff pt who had miscarried fetus O/N and had since left hospital. Fetus at 19.2 weeks. Policy re handling fetus consulted. Night staff stated they offered pt to see fetus. Declined, said she just wanted to leave and did so. Discussed pt emotional support w/ staff. Plan: RN to phone pt during shift and offer another chance to see the fetus. If yes, prepare fetus for pt viewing. Appropriate and respectful fetal disposal.

When I was at this placement, D/W was an accepted shorthand for ‘Discussed with’ and O/N was an accepted shorthand for ‘Overnight’, or ‘during the night’.

This clinical note outlines that the night shift staff were consulted in relation to how to best care for the patient, even though she was no longer in the hospital. It notes the fetal age and that the policy related to handling miscarriages was consulted. It further records that night staff had offered the patient to see the fetus and the patient's response and subsequent departure. It notes that the patient's emotional support was discussed. It records the plan to contact the patient and ask her again if she wanted to view the fetus and what to do if she said yes. Lastly, and very importantly, it notes that the fetal body was to be respectfully disposed of in the appropriate manner. As it turned out, this was a good plan as when the patient was contacted after having had some time to recover and consider what had happened, she did want to see her baby. The plan was enacted appropriately and the best result that could be achieved in such a circumstance was.

The key concept is that incidental nursing care may not involve equipment or procedures, but it remains essential nursing work. When documenting such care, record the essence of what occurred, avoid unnecessary quotation, and ensure meaningful actions are not omitted.

Incidental nursing care informs future planning and contributes directly to the overall nursing care plan. It reflects the human side of nursing, often shaping how patients remember their care. Documenting incidental care with the same professionalism as procedures is a hallmark of good nursing practice.

Chapter 9: The Nursing Care Plan

Planning Is Not the Nursing Care Plan

By this point in the book, we have spoken about the patient encounter, specific nursing tasks, disruptive care events, concluding the encounter, and planning future care. It is important now to clarify how planning and the nursing care plan relate to each other — because they are not the same thing, although they are closely connected.

Earlier, we discussed writing a plan at the end of a nursing entry. That plan reflects short-term, practical intent:

- What needs to happen next
- What tasks remain
- What orders need to be followed up

The nursing care plan, by contrast, is broader, slower, and more conceptual. It is not tied to a single encounter or shift. It describes why care is being given, what the care goals are, and how nursing interventions support those goals over time. This is the plan that my American ex-Navy

Nursing Tutor was referring to. A good nurse should be able to relate the basics of the nursing care plan to the patient - or at least where the patient is at within the nursing care plan - and the steps they were taking to accomplish it today. Those 'today' steps refer to the plan the individual nurse has for caring for the patient in the here and now.

In simple terms:

- The nursing care plan answers: Why are we doing this?
- Your plan answers: What am I doing next?

Why Nursing Care Plans Matter (Even When They Feel Abstract)

Many student nurses struggle with nursing care plans. They can feel artificial, repetitive, or disconnected from real patient care. This feeling is understandable, especially when the pressure of the shift demands practical action rather than theoretical structure.

However, the nursing care plan serves an important purpose. It:

- Provides a shared understanding of the patient's problems and needs
- Aligns nursing care across multiple shifts and staff
- Prevents care from becoming fragmented or task-driven
- Encourages nurses to think holistically

A good nursing care plan keeps the patient from becoming a collection of isolated tasks. It reminds us that wound care, observations, education, and comfort measures are all part of a single therapeutic story.

How the Nursing Care Plan Connects to the Patient Encounter

Every patient encounter you document contributes to the nursing care plan, whether you explicitly realise it or not.

When you perform wound care, manage pain, educate a patient, respond to a disruptive care event or adjust future plans, you are either:

- Progressing the nursing care plan, or
- Revealing that the nursing care plan needs review

Examples of this include:

- A well healing wound confirms that the current plan is effective
- A wound that deteriorates suggests the plan needs to change
- A patient who refuses care requires reassessment of goals and approach

Therefore, the nursing care plan is not static. It evolves through patient encounters.

Who Owns the Nursing Care Plan?

Although nursing care plans are often initiated on admission, every nurse contributes to them.

You do not need to write a brand-new nursing care plan every shift. What you do need to do is:

- Understand the existing nursing care plan
- Ensure your care aligns with it
- Update it when the patient's needs change

If you notice that what you are doing bears little resemblance to what is written in the nursing care plan, that is a signal that something needs review.

The Nursing Care Plan Beyond the Encounter

In many settings, particularly community health and chronic disease management, the nursing care plan forms part of the patient's referral. It may be included formally in written documentation or communicated through structured handover.

This means that the nursing care plan does not only guide care within one ward or service. It often shapes how care is delivered across settings and by other professionals. A clear, thoughtful nursing care plan helps ensure that when a patient moves between services, the intent of care moves with them.

Nursing Care Plans and Medical Orders

It is important to distinguish between:

- Medical orders (what doctors prescribe), and
- Nursing care plans (how nursing care supports recovery)

Doctors diagnose and prescribe. Nurses assess, plan, implement, and evaluate care. While medical orders inform nursing care, they do not replace nursing judgement.

For example, a doctor may order antibiotics, while a nurse plans wound care, monitors response, educates the patient, and escalates concerns. In this way, the nursing care plan sits alongside medical management, not beneath it.

Nursing Care Plans Across Settings

The complexity of a nursing care plan will vary by setting.

In acute care, Nursing Care Plans may be brief and problem focused. They may change rapidly. They are closely linked to immediate medical treatment. However, in community and chronic care, nursing care plans are often longer-term. They focus on function, independence, quality of life and education. They also often require coordination with external healthcare services.

Regardless of setting, the principles remain the same: assess, plan, implement and evaluate. Rinse and repeat.

Linking It All Together

By now, you should be able to see how each part of the nursing process fits together:

- The initial patient encounter assesses the need for immediate medical attention and establishes context.
- Specific nursing tasks deliver needed therapeutic care
- Disruptive care events test nursing clinical judgement during the patient encounter.
- Concluding the encounter ensures closure and reassures the patient
- The plan sets the immediate nursing care direction.
- Incidental Nursing Care involves tasks carried out that also help the patient achieve their health goals
- The nursing care plan provides the overarching framework within which nursing care takes place.

None of these exist in isolation. Good nursing care flows between them.

A Reassuring Final Note for Student Nurses

If nursing care planning feels difficult at first, you are not alone. It improves with experience, reflection, and repeated patient encounters. Often, it will be established before being handed over to you. That said, if you can answer these questions in relation to your patient, you are already thinking like a nurse:

- Does this patient need immediate medical attention?
- If not, what does this patient need right now?
- What are we trying to accomplish?
- What might get in the way?
- What happens next?

The nursing care plan is simply a structured way of recording those answers. Your individual plan that you record after each patient encounter reflects the tasks you and other nurses are going to do to work towards accomplishing the nursing care plan.

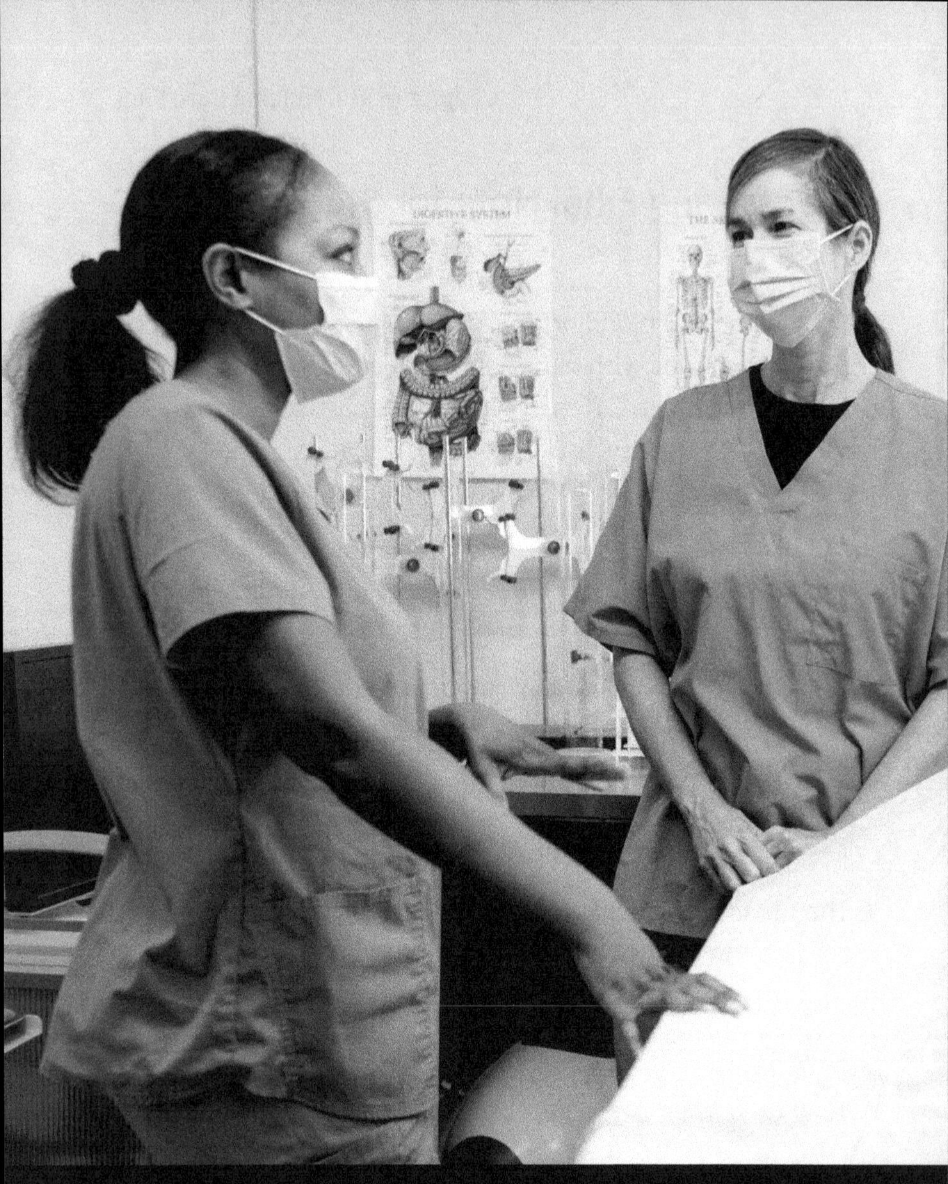

Do all you can to foster a positive work environment. Be patient with your colleagues. Remember that we are all in this together.

Case Studies

The following case studies are full examples of how I would document certain encounters putting everything together that has been discussed. They do not reflect the only way to record nursing encounters, but they do reflect the overall patient encounter as explained in this book. Remember that whatever is documented here, local health policies and procedures must be followed. Please do not look so much at the substance of what is written. Instead focus on how the overall encounter is recorded.

Please also be aware that, in these examples, the patient notes are not necessarily written at one moment at the end of the day. They are meant to be documented as they occur, or as soon as possible after the event.

Case Study 1:

A patient is handed over at the 7:00am shift. The patient is recovering from pneumonia and is on Twice Daily oral antibiotics for that illness. She also has other medication prescribed that she needs to take. There is a MO order for imaging for the patient, a chest x-ray. The following records only the nurse's notes over the shift.

0720	Pt handed over at 0700 from RN Brown. Resting in bed. Alert + oriented. Normal breathing. No pain. Mood is good. Attending to ADLs. O/E: Pt on active monitoring. Pt on O2 via nasal prongs at 2L PRN. Obs as charted. Within acceptable parameters. Plan: BD obs. For ABs and meds as charted. Organise imaging. For routine personal care.
0730	0730: ABs and meds as charted. No issues noted or raised.
0825	Pt ate breakfast. No issues noted or raised.
0918	Organised pt's appointment with imaging as per MO order. Pt for PM imaging. Pt informed of same.

0955	Routine personal care attended to. Pt self-mobilised to shower. Self-caring. RTB. Monitoring equipment and O2 reconnected. No issues noted or raised.
1236	Pt ate lunch. No issues noted or raised.
1300	Imaging arrived to collect pt. Escorted pt to imaging w/ portable O2 2L via nasal prongs.
1332	RTW. Pt reconnected to O2. All monitoring leads reattached. Pt resting comfortably. No issues raised or noted.
1400	Pt handed over to RN Johns. No issues raised or noted.

Case Study 2:

In this case study, the patient is a community health patient who is receiving wound care at the local health clinic. In community health, unless an issue is raised, one entry per patient per visit happens.

Pt attended clinic. Alert + oriented. Normal breathing. No pain. Mood is good. Attending to ADLs.

For wound care.

Previous dressings removed.

Small amount of purulent exudate on previous dressings. Some strikethrough noted.

O/E:

The wound measures 7 cm x 3 cm. Approximately 0.5 cm depth. Pink granulating tissue. Small amount of yellow slough on wound bed. No signs or symptoms of infection. Peri wound the skin is healthy and intact.

Procedure:

Washed with normal saline

Betadine to wound bed

Zetuvit 10x10 to cover

Mefix to secure

Pt requested earlier apt at 8:00am on Friday as she will be out that morning. Time unavailable. Offered 2:15pm to give the pt time to get home. Pt happy with this time. Appointment reminder given.

Pt happy with service. No complaints voiced.

Plan:

Pt for Twice Weekly wound care (Tues/Fri)

Next appointment Friday 23/01/2026 at 2:15pm.

Case Study 3:

This case study is for IVAB administration as commonly occurs in Hospital In the Home settings. Here, a patient is receiving IVABs once per day at home.

AIDH refers to the Australian Injectables Drugs Handbook. This book contains the instructions on how to prepare medications for IV administration. Please check your local health service policies for the equivalent manual.

> Pt home for visit. Alert + oriented. Normal breathing. No pain. Mood is good. Attending to ADLs.
>
> For daily IVABs.
>
> O/E:
>
> There is a 18 Fr cannula located in the pt's right forearm. Dressings intact.
>
> No signs or symptoms of infection.
>
> Procedure:
>
> Carried out using ANTT.
>
> Pt verified using medication order and consent obtained.
>
> Bung swabbed with chlorhex.
>
> 10 ml NS flush. Line patent.
>
> IVABs administered as per AIDH guidelines.
>
> 10 ml NS flush.

Obs taken. Within acceptable parameters.

Pain nil.

Pt aware of IVAB visit tomorrow morning. No issues raised or noted.

Pt happy with service. No complaints voiced.

Plan:

IVABs to continue.

Next appointment 20/1/2026 AM.

Closing Reflection

Good nursing is not only about completing tasks. It is about understanding the patient's journey, where they are at in their journey and contributing meaningfully to that journey. The overarching goal is to help people be able to complete activities of daily living without the need for extra help or in a way that doesn't tax them so heavily that other aspects of an enjoyable life are not so greatly impacted. The nursing care plan exists to support that understanding for you, for your colleagues, and most importantly, for the patient. Your role is to care enough to help where you can and to ask for help when a task exceeds your current skill levels. Asking for help is not weakness. In nursing, it can be a lifesaving sign of strength.

Good nursing is also rarely about doing more. It is about doing what is needed, documenting it clearly, and leaving the patient — and the next nurse — in the best possible position.

I sincerely hope that through good nursing care - and through good documentation of that care - you discover the joy and satisfaction that comes from helping someone through a vulnerable time in their lives. It is truly a rewarding experience.

About the Author

Daniel Moir became a nurse later in life, earning a Bachelor of Nursing from the University of Canberra. In 2012, he undertook his nursing graduate year at Queanbeyan District Hospital in New South Wales, Australia. After completing his graduate year, he secured a position as a community nurse at Queanbeyan Hospital, where he later became the Community Health Clinical Nurse Educator.

He subsequently moved with his wife and children to Camden, NSW, where he worked within the South Western Sydney Local Health District as a Clinical Nurse Educator.

In 2020, he commenced a Graduate Law degree with the University of Canberra. In December 2022, with one assignment remaining before completing his degree, he was hospitalised and diagnosed with a subarachnoid haemorrhage, subsequent severe vasospasm, and hydrocephalus. Ongoing health complications have meant he has been unable to return to nursing or pursue a career in law.

In this book, he channels the insight gained from his time as a Clinical Nurse Educator into guiding and supporting new nurses and health professionals as they begin their professional journeys.

www.ingramcontent.com/pod-product-compliance
Lightning Source LLC
LaVergne TN
LVHW010735061126
851857LV00014B/1497
* 9 7 8 1 7 6 4 2 2 5 6 4 9 *